Welcome to Alopecia

NITKA MARGA

First Edition

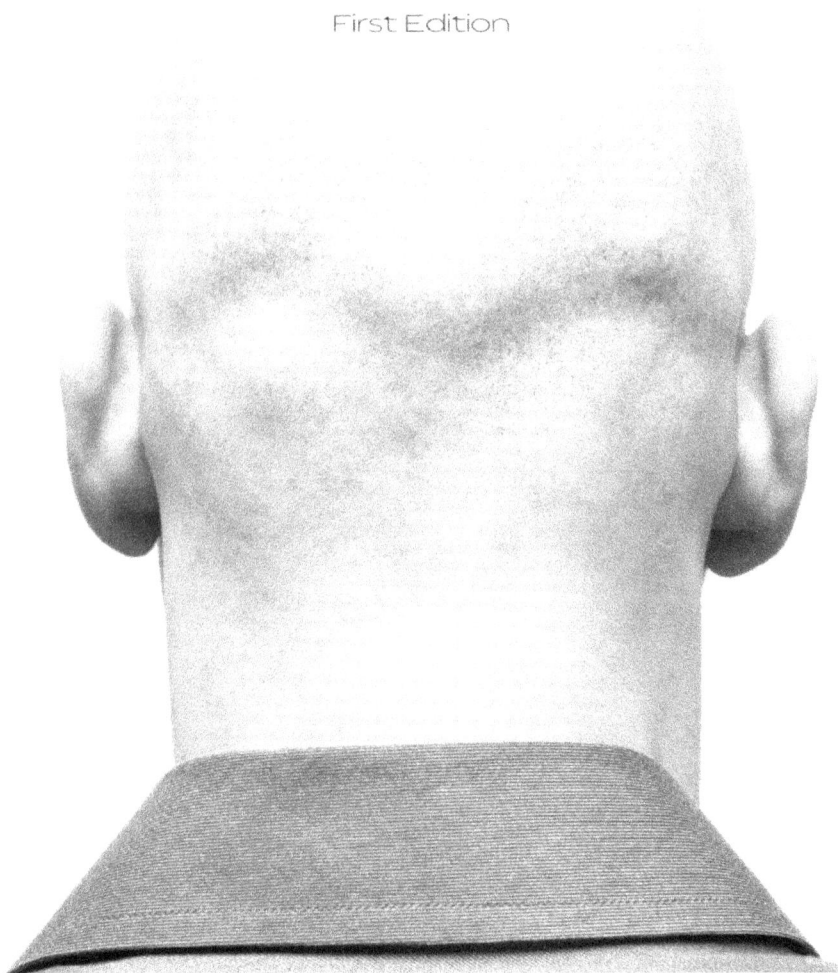

Welcome to Alopecia

By Nitka Marga

Published by SoulBound Books, 2023

Printed by Amazon KDP

Cover Creation: SoulBound Books

Elements of cover and images created using Canva.

ISBN: **979-8-9891265-2-1**

www.SoulBoundBooksinfo.com

Welcome to Alopecia
NITKA MARGA

Contents

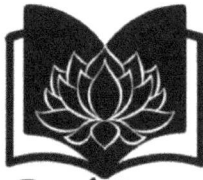

SoulBound
BOOKS

Forward

Welcome to the inaugural edition of "Welcome to Alopecia." This is more than just a book; it's a heartfelt journey woven with personal insights, lessons, and moments from my experience with alopecia. My intention is not merely to share my narrative but to ignite a sense of solace, self-acceptance, and empowerment in those navigating similar paths.

As life's journey is perpetual, so too will this narrative evolve. I envision a Second Edition that will be enriched not only by my own growth as an individual and an author but also by the invaluable contributions from you, the reader. I wholeheartedly encourage feedback, reviews, and personal testimonials about alopecia so that future iterations can be even more resonant and impactful.

While centered around alopecia, the essence of this book transcends its specific subject matter. It speaks to the heart of vulnerability and the universality of our human experiences. Whether you're confronting alopecia or any other challenge that calls for courage, understanding, and compassion, I invite you to find solace and strength within these pages.

Welcome to our shared journey.

A Note on the Quotes Ahead:

In the following pages, you'll find quotes from individuals whose lives were marked by profound challenges, adversities, and achievements. Their resilience in the face of such trials stands as a testament to the indomitable spirit of humanity.

It's essential to recognize that the trials and tribulations of living with alopecia, though deeply personal and often challenging, differ significantly from the life-altering events faced by some of the quoted figures. By including their words, we in no way equate the struggles of alopecia with their profound experiences. However, the essence of their wisdom—resilience, hope, courage, and empowerment—speaks to universal truths that transcend specifics.

Feelings are, in many ways, a relative landscape. Each individual's pain, joy, sorrow, and happiness are genuine, valid, and felt deeply. While alopecia might seem insignificant in comparison to the vast historical challenges, to those experiencing it, the emotions are every bit as real.

Let these quotes serve as an inspiration. Not just because of the words themselves, but due to the lives and stories behind them. May they remind you that resilience is possible, hope is always present, and that you are never alone in your journey.

"You may not control all the events that happen to you, but you can decide not to be reduced by them."

Maya Angelou

Embracing the Bald Truth

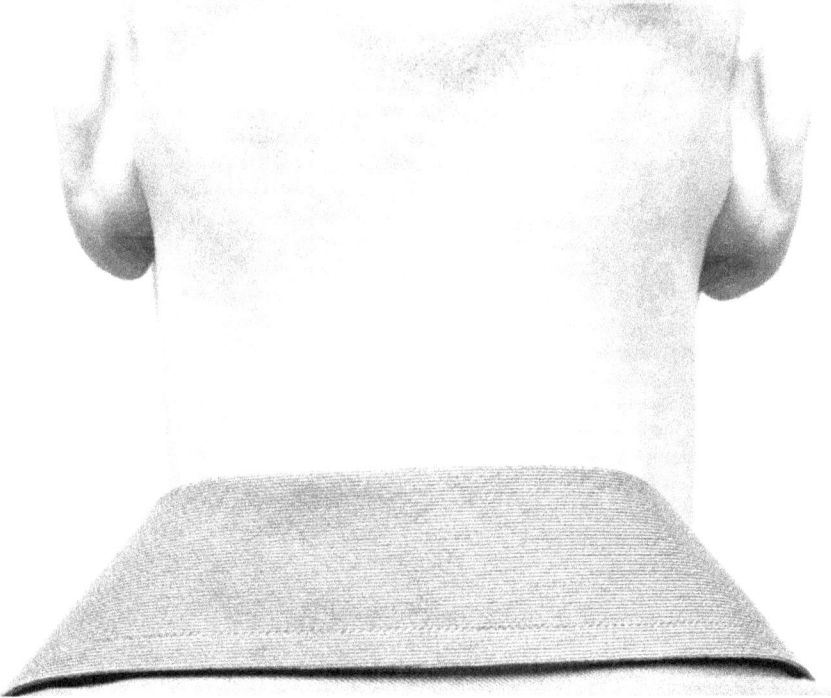

If you're here thinking I'm going to offer a comforting pat on the back or a story sprinkled with roses and rainbows, you might as well close the book right now. This is about Alopecia—my story, your story, our journey. No fluff, just the raw, unfiltered truth.

I was a freshman in high school when my hair decided it had better places to be. Now, age 33, my head, lashes, and brows are barren landscapes. Now, you might think I'd say, "Losing my hair didn't change the core of who I am, only my looks."

Not True! No, I won't feed you that line.

It transformed me back then and continues to shape me now.

I've heard the comforting whispers, the soothing words from well-meaning souls: "It only changes who you are on the outside, not the inside." Says someone who hasn't seen their reflection morph so dramatically. Imagine a future where your hair is a distant memory. Life doesn't just go on as usual. I've walked this path, and in a twist of fate, I'm genuinely grateful for it. Sounds strange, but losing my hair at a young age might have been a gift in a brutal disguise.

Our journey starts at the truth. The raw, unvarnished. If you're teetering on the edge of hair loss, knee-deep in it, or have journeyed through its entirety, your truth right now might be, "**This sucks.**" And that's valid.

I'm not a doctor or therapist, and this isn't a prescription. I'm a yoga enthusiast, an entrepreneur, and I ride the highs and lows of life. I've faced hair loss at a young age, and as tumultuous as it was, it might've been my most profound teacher.

Welcome to the world of hair loss. I don't have sympathy for you. But I have a ton of **empathy**.

Chapter 1

Sympathy Isn't What You Need

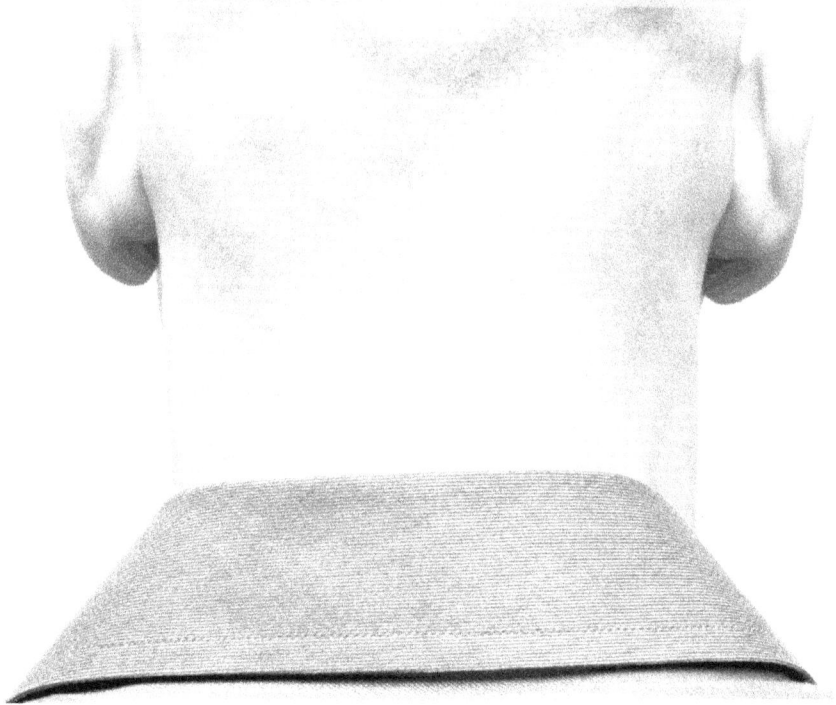

First off, if you're looking for sympathy, you won't find it here. Surprised? Good, stick with me.

I've been served up a fair share of "Be grateful for what you have" and "It's only hair; the real you remains unchanged." Honestly, if I banked a dollar every time these clichés got thrown at me, I'd be the proud owner of a hair transplant empire. But let's cut the crap: that's sympathy. And sympathy? It's a lousy substitute for understanding.

What we're really chasing is raw, unvarnished empathy. That unapologetic truth that only comes from someone who's been in the trenches. Losing your hair? Trust me, it's a gut punch. Spotted a bald patch on your beard? That's another low blow. When you get those reality checks, that sinking feeling? It's you facing the facts, no filter.

Here's the cold, hard truth: Alopecia isn't just about your looks; it reshapes you. Not just your appearance, but your mind, your emotions, how you perceive the world. It's going to drag you through the mud, challenge every ounce of your being, and then, after all the turmoil, it's going to gift you something profound. A vulnerability, a strength, and a resilience you might not know you have.

It's a twisted gift, but a gift nonetheless.

So, here's where we stand, staring down this path. Alopecia isn't the apocalypse, but don't kid yourself—it's no picnic either. It's a journey. And I'm here, committing to call it as I see it. I'm not here to coddle you with fluffy sentiments, but to say, "This is hard, we are stronger

—

6

than we know." It's not about empty sympathy; it's about vulnerability, empathy, and in-turn, genuine connection with yourself, and with others.

Embracing vulnerability provides a unique kind of power. When we let our guard down, when we show our scars and not just our triumphs, we connect on a level that's real and profound. It's a universal language, one that speaks of shared struggles and resilience.

For those losing all or most of their hair, this vulnerability is on full display. Every day, every moment—**it's there for the world to see**. While some can hide their vulnerabilities, tuck them away behind masks and pretenses, yours is out in the open. There might be moments where you wish to hide, to shield the world from your truth, but that choice isn't always at your disposal. And it's in this exposure, in this raw openness, where true strength is forged.

Wearing your vulnerability so openly may feel daunting and overwhelming. But remember, it also means you're facing the world with profound courage. Every glance, every whispered comment, every unspoken judgment—they're all challenges you confront head-on (pun intended). Where others may have the luxury of hiding, you stand unyielding, your vulnerability both your challenge and your emblem of resilience.

I still remember the day I found that first bald spot. It felt like the world had thrown a curveball, aiming right for my gut. But here's the reality of Alopecia: it doesn't just rob you of hair. It shaves layers off your self-esteem, holds a mirror up to your vulnerabilities, and then, after tearing you down, it forces you to rebuild. The process is agonizing, but the transformation; it's profound. It's like forging steel – heated, hammered, and then emerging stronger than ever.

If you're looking for a companion on this tumultuous journey, you've found one. I won't sugar-coat or offer shallow comforts. I'll be the voice that says, "This is a nightmare, but you're not alone."

It's not about misplaced sympathy; it's about shared pain, resilience, and genuine empathy.

Your first assignment? Walk up to a mirror, meet your reflection head-on, and let everything out. This isn't just about confronting your new look; it's about honesty, it's about empathy, it's about connection. Don't censor your emotions; let them flow. Raw. Real. Unfiltered. This confrontation, as unsettling as it may be, is our starting line. It's where we dig deep, where we grow, and where we find the strength to rewrite the narrative of beauty on our own terms.

Again, welcome. And thank you for existing. I wrote this for you because **you're awesome.** I tip my hat and my shiny head to you.

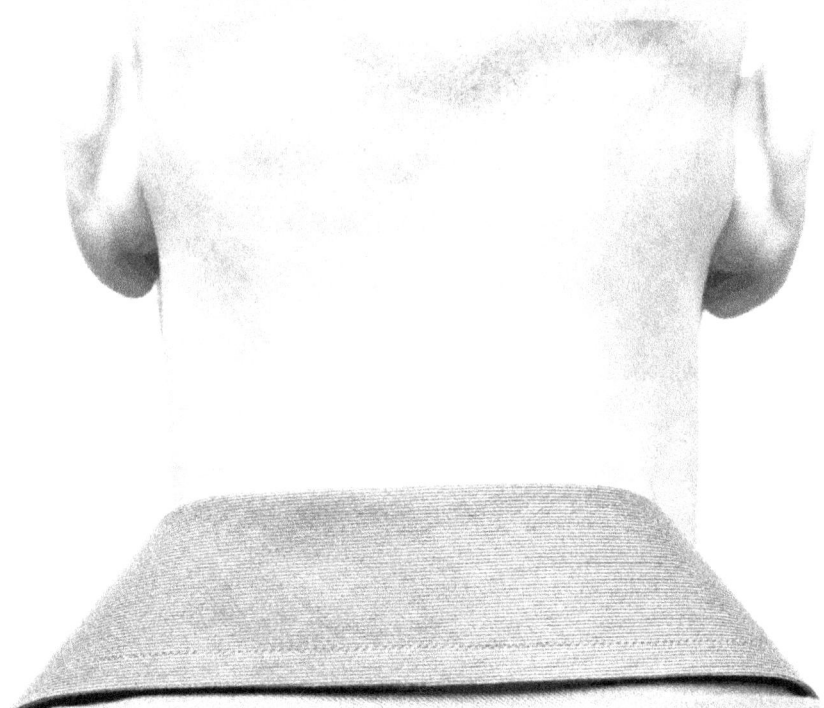

Chapter 2

Let's Talk About 'You'

When I use the word 'you,' I'm not alluding to the divine self, to the absence of ego, the embrace of it, or anything remotely philosophical in that sense. And yes, I sense some raised eyebrows because, as a yoga teacher and an eternal student, I often find myself enveloped in delightful discussions about eastern philosophies.

Here, when I talk about 'you', I'm pointing straight to you. The tangible you—your body, your mind, your swirling emotions, your rampant thoughts, your deepest feelings. That's the 'you' this narrative will address.

As a mediator I would love to dive into the idea that you are not your thoughts, but that's for a different time.

You are you – a marvel. Yes, **you**.

You are a complex being, and a miracle. The intricacies of your body are unfathomably dynamic.

For a moment, consider the countless books penned, experiments conducted, and hours dedicated to unraveling the mysteries that reside within you.

Here, we are, with hearts that pump, lungs that breathe, and minds that think, all without asking them to do so… I mean, come on? It's wildly incredible when we think about it - our bodies, these complex machines of flesh, blood and water.

This moment is a salute, a toast if you will, to the phenomenal wonder of our existence in this precise moment. **Whether crowned with hair or not.**

Standing amid our vast universe, have you ever taken a moment to truly salute the human body? To stand in sheer awe of its grandeur, its intricacies, and even its imperfections? The heart that races during a chase, the hands that shake in anticipation, the eyes that well up at poignant memories—all of it, a testament to the marvel that is you.

Yet, the beautiful reality of 'you' is that you are always in flux, just like the meandering river. It twists, it turns, it surges with power and retreats in tranquility. It's ceaselessly shaping and reshaping its course, but at its essence, it remains pure, unchanging water. This fluidity, this adaptability, is what you embody.

Jet Li once said, **"Be like water."** And that's precisely the state of being we're striving for. Because in life, there will be moments that reshape us. Losing your hair is one of those moments. It will sculpt your course, and it grants you a unique power: the power to steer that change, to determine its depth and direction.

Now, here's a universal truth: change is not exclusive to hair loss. Remember Darwin's wisdom:

"It is not the strongest of the species that survives, nor the most intelligent; it is the one most adaptable to change."

If you're a young reader navigating the tricky waters of hair loss, first off, kudos to you. And kudos to your badass parents for letting you read a book peppered with some intense vocabulary! Seriously, when I say, "**You're an awesome badass**," trust me, I mean every word. But on a deeper note, understand this: **change is inevitable**. And I'm not merely referring to the superficial transitions, like getting taller, developing wrinkles, or losing more hair (if that's a possibility).

The essence of our existence is in constant motion. Much like the river's water, we have the gift of carving our own path, of defining our journey. And if there's anything life has taught me, it's that our ability to adapt, to "be the water," only sharpens with adversity.

So, yes, I maintain my stance. I won't sugarcoat this journey for you. It's hard, it's messy, and sometimes, it feels downright unfair. But remember: you are a marvel, and you are the river. Embrace your fluidity, navigate the rapids, and I promise, the ride won't just be about survival; **it'll be one hell of an exhilarating journey.**

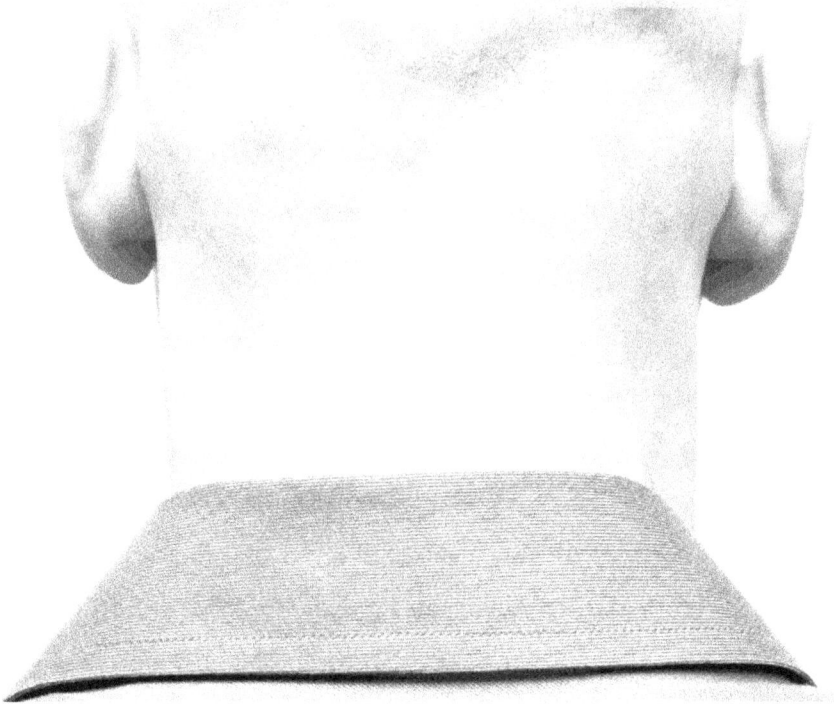

Chapter 3

The Symphony of Life

At first glance, you might wonder how we've taken a detour from hair and self-identity to the realm of **music**. But bear with me. This isn't a detour; **it's an integral part of the journey.** As we navigate the challenges of alopecia, we need a companion, a salve for our wounds, a melody to guide our steps. And that's precisely where music comes into play.

Music, in its essence, is the language of the soul. It's not only a collection of sounds and rhythms but a bridge between the most profound parts of our beings and the world around us. It has the power to capture emotions that words often fail to convey. The joy of a new beginning, the sorrow of a painful ending, the anticipation of what's to come—**all encapsulated in notes and harmonies.**

Think about those times when you've been at a loss for words, when emotions seemed too complex to articulate. Now, imagine finding a song that speaks to your soul, encapsulating those feelings with uncanny accuracy. Music has that unparalleled ability—**to give voice to our deepest sentiments when words fall short.** It's a source of solace, a wellspring of joy, a catalyst for catharsis. In the ups and downs of life, especially as you navigate the challenges of alopecia, music offers a comforting constant, like a steadfast friend who knows just what to say.

As you grapple with the changes alopecia brings, let music be your anchor. Let it remind you of the harmony that exists even when life seems out of tune. It can be a song from your childhood that brings a smile to your face, a ballad that echoes your current struggles, or an anthem that empowers you to keep pushing forward. Music is an elixir, a healer, a friend that understands even when no one else does.

I urge you to find solace in music, to let it fill the gaps and spaces as you traverse this journey. Play it loud when you need to scream to the world, softly when you seek a moment of introspection, or on repeat when you find a song that speaks to your soul. Because, amidst the silence of our struggles, it's the symphony of music that often speaks the loudest.

Next time you find yourself overwhelmed or lost, put on those headphones or turn up the speakers. Let the rhythms, melodies, and lyrics cradle you, guide you, and remind you of the ever-present beauty and strength within you. Dive into the world of music and discover yet another facet of the incredible tapestry that is 'you.'

Shifting our focus now, we glide from the comforting embrace of melodies to the glitz and glam of the big screen. Ah, the world of movie stars and TV icons—do any of them proudly showcase their alopecia-ridden scalps? I immediately think of Bruce Willis with his iconic rugged charm and Dwayne "The Rock" Johnson, with a baldness that's become almost as famous as his towering biceps. But do they truly represent the alopecia community? Maybe not in the strictest sense.

Pause for a second. Let me delve deep into my almost two-decade-long archive of hairless memories. There must be someone else who boldly represents the alopecia community in the world of celluloid.

...I'm back... And I missed you.

Well, while Hollywood may be sparse with alopecian ambassadors, I did find a few who've been open about their hair battles. But none truly stand tall as the face of alopecia. My sincere apologies if I've missed out on any shining beacon in this regard.

It's striking, isn't it? Flick through channels or skim through the latest movie trailers, and you'd be hard-pressed to find those like us represented. It's not a blame game. We are, after all, a minority. And truth be told, I don't feel slighted. But what's imperative is acknowledging this absence. The lack of hairless figures on TV, in movies, even on billboards—it signifies something.

Whether this omission stems from market dynamics, beauty standards, or just pure coincidence, the effect it has is clear. It makes us feel unique, isolated, and starkly different. It's not about a revolution to change what we see. It's about understanding and recognizing the feeling it evokes, especially for someone who's in the tumultuous phase of rapidly losing hair.

We're not seeking a seat at every table or a representation quota. We're asking for understanding, for empathy. We want the world to know that yes, it feels different when our own image doesn't reflect back from the cultural mirrors around us. But through it all, we find strength. We find unity in our community. And in this journey of understanding and acceptance, we realize the profound truth: sometimes, the most impactful stories are the ones told off-screen.

For now, I'm going to let the soothing tunes of Coldplay wash over me. See you in the next chapter, and thanks for sticking with me. Through the highs, lows, and silent gaps, remember:

We're in this together, even when we're timelines apart.

Chapter 4

From Solitude to Spotlight

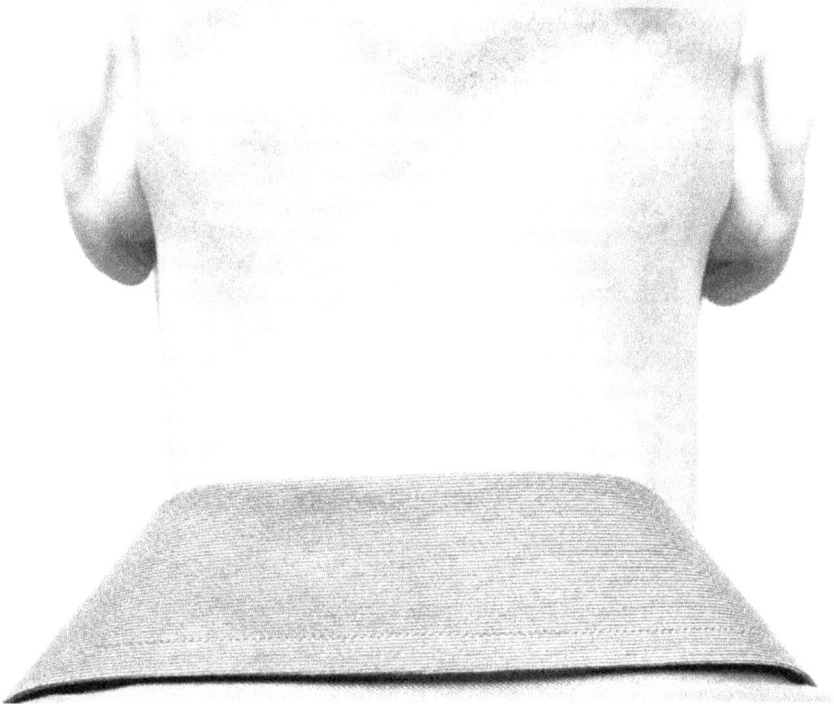

The sunlight filtered weakly through the curtains, casting muted patterns on the walls. The droning hum of "Free Bird" blasted from the speakers, as my fingers flew across the plastic buttons of the Guitar Hero controller. With each note, I felt a momentary reprieve, a fleeting escape from the suffocating weight of my reality.

For over a week, this dimly lit room had been both my refuge and prison. Time seemed to blur, with days melding into nights. The world outside held little appeal, fading into insignificance. The weight in my chest wasn't just heavy; it was crushing. Every heartbeat echoed the raw, glaring truth: I was bald.

It wasn't a choice, nor a fashion-forward declaration. It was a desperate act. A final capitulation to the relentless alopecia that had, over months, turned my once-lustrous dirty blonde hair into an inconsistent canvas of skin. One emotionally charged day, I couldn't stomach the sight any longer, and I took to it with clippers. Each falling strand felt like shards of my identity being cruelly sheared off.

My sanctuary was this room, the melodies of Guitar Hero, and the obscurity provided by dim lighting. But one grim morning, that sanctuary was invaded when my parents decreed it was time. No sugar-coated words, no comforting assurances. "You're going back to school," they stated unequivocally. The very thought sent tremors of anxiety through me. How could I face the world, especially the unforgiving hallways of high school, looking like this?

Whispers had reached me, even in my seclusion. The news of my drastic 'transformation' had spread like wildfire. Teachers, staff, classmates — everyone seemed to know. My intensely personal struggle had become a topic of public discourse. Though the intention might have been one of compassion, to my ears, it dripped with pity. The last thing I yearned for was to become a spectacle or, worse yet, a living lesson in 'resilience'.

Yet, as the clock continued its relentless march, I was confronted with an inescapable realization: my room, despite its comforting shadows and the distraction of the game, was not a permanent solution.

This desire to hide, to cocoon myself from the world's piercing gaze, wasn't unique to this incident. As I grew older, I would discover that there were other facets of life, other challenges, that would push me into similar corners of despair. But that is a tale for another time…

The stillness of the empty hallways was haunting as I entered the school late. **It felt like stepping onto a stage, under the brightest spotlight, with an audience you couldn't see.** As an office staff member escorted me to my first class, every step seemed to amplify the thundering heartbeat in my ears. The anticipation, the fear, the crushing weight of uncertainty – it was all-consuming.
I braced myself for the stares, the whispers, and the silent judgments. But as the door swung open, revealing a room full of familiar faces, I was met with something unexpected: a mixture of surprise, curiosity, and simple smiles.

Sure, there were hushed murmurs and some stolen glances, but the apocalypse I had imagined never came. Was I anxious? Beyond words. Did it hurt? Hell yes, every single moment of it. Did I want my hair back? Of course! But honestly…

The reality wasn't as horrific as the monsters I had conjured in my mind.

Indeed, there will always be that small percentage, the ones who use cruelty as a shield against their own insecurities. There were snide remarks and underhanded comments. But such voices were, surprisingly, in the minority. Most people, I found, were intrinsically kind. They extended understanding, offered smiles, and slowly, the vast chasm of fear I had created in my mind began to narrow.

Days turned to weeks, and weeks to months. And with time, a realization dawned – my baldness, which I once viewed as a crippling flaw, had become a unique signature. It was a badge of individuality in a sea of conformity. By the time I was preparing to bid farewell to high school, it was clear that this 'uniqueness' had its silver linings. Almost everyone knew me, not just for my appearance, but for the person I was. And the truth is, I relished the attention. Not because I was vain, but because it opened doors to countless friendships and interactions.

Looking back, the taunts and jibes were but fleeting shadows. They paled in comparison to the warmth, acceptance, and camaraderie I felt. People, for the most part, are kind-hearted. And as I navigated this tumultuous chapter, I was reminded of an essential truth:

Sometimes, our fears and insecurities loom larger than life, and the reality can be much kinder than we anticipate.

To those of you reading this, who might be grappling with a similar challenge or any challenge that's urging you to hide away:

Firstly, let me make something clear. I don't offer you my sympathy. Sympathy often comes from a place of pity, and **I genuinely believe you don't need pity**. What you need is understanding, acknowledgment, and perhaps a gentle push.

Go to school. Step out into the world. Face those demons, confront those fears. Yes, it might suck — it really might. The anxiety, the uncertainty, the self-consciousness, they're all real and palpable. I've been there. And here's the catch:

Even when it's hard, even when it's excruciating, it will be worth it.

Every challenge, every discomfort, every snide remark or curious gaze you endure – they all contribute to a stronger, more resilient version of you. **Every time you stand up to face another day, despite the**

weight in your heart, you're writing a chapter of courage in your life story.

Because here's the truth: hiding away might offer temporary comfort, but it's out there, amidst the chaos, the judgments, and the love, that we truly grow. And trust me when I say this — in the grand tapestry of your life, these challenges will just be threads that add depth and texture to your story.

So, chin up. Embrace the world with all its imperfections and remember: even in the toughest moments, there's an opportunity, a lesson, a silver lining. Go out and find it. It's waiting for you, and believe me, **it will all be worth it.**

Chapter 5

The Stress Paradox

The day I was diagnosed with Alopecia, I remember the doctor's face. Calm, empathetic, with a hint of professional detachment. His words, intended to be reassuring, still ring in my ears, "Try not to stress over it." A simple statement, yet packed with such profound irony. It was as if someone had just told me not to think of a pink elephant. Naturally, the only thing I could think of was a pink elephant. Or in this case, the all-consuming stress of rapidly losing my hair.

Stress, as science tells us, is both a cause and a consequence of autoimmune diseases. It's a classic chicken-and-egg situation. Does the disease cause stress or does stress exacerbate the disease? The more I mulled over it, the more entangled I became in this web of causality.

As the days turned into months and years, a more significant realization dawned upon me: **perhaps it wasn't about avoiding stress but about dealing with it**. After all, stress is an inevitable part of life, be it from external factors like work and relationships or internal battles like health and self-worth.

Over the years, I've come to see stress not as an enemy but as a messenger. It's a signal from our body and mind, urging us to take a step back, to recalibrate and reassess. Instead of drowning in it, I began to search for ways to navigate its tumultuous waters.

1. **Acceptance Over Resistance:**
   The first step in my journey was to stop resisting. The more I fought the stress, the stronger it grew. Accepting it, acknowledging its presence, was liberating. It didn't make the stress disappear, but it prevented it from becoming a monstrous entity in my mind.

2. **Mindfulness and Meditation:**
   I delved into the world of meditation. The act of simply being, of focusing on the present moment, anchored me. Those fleeting moments of tranquility became my oasis in the desert of chaos.

3. **Seeking Support:**
   Talking helped. Whether it was with close friends, family, or therapist, vocalizing my fears and anxieties lifted some of the burdens. In the shared experiences of others and support, I found solace and understanding.

4. **Channeling It Creatively:**

   I took up journaling. Pouring my feelings onto paper was therapeutic. Some days, it was a stream of consciousness; other days, structured narratives. It became an outlet, a way to process and release pent-up emotions. My passion for writing was born out of introspective journaling. Fast forward nearly two decades, I've written about six books. I've published two comedies and I'm currently preparing to publish my third book. This one will be about welcoming you to alopecia... Welcome!

5. **Physical Activity:**

   Moving my body, whether it was a brisk walk, a run, or just simple stretches, helped dispel the nervous energy. The endorphins, rightfully termed 'feel-good chemicals,' did their magic. As my journey continued, I discover yoga. Since then, I have taught over 2500 classes, and have no plans on stopping.

Over time, I learned that while I couldn't control the external triggers of stress, I had a say in how I responded to it. The journey isn't linear. There were days I felt overwhelmed, but each moment of despair was met with an equally powerful moment of resilience.

The doctor's advice, though initially perplexing, was a gateway. It thrust me into a journey of self-discovery, pushing me to find ways to cope, adapt, and thrive. To anyone grappling with stress, know this:

It's not about eradicating stress from your life; it's about forging a relationship with it.

Understanding stress, mold it, use it as a catalyst for growth. For in the heart of stress lies not just discomfort but also the potential for unparalleled growth and evolution.

Remember, amidst life's challenges, the ability to dance in the rain, to find joy in adversity, rests within you. Harness it, and let it guide you through the storms and into the dawn of a new day.

As for the days where stress holds you down and resilience momentarily retreats, know that **you are human**. You have been gifted with a wide variety of thoughts, feelings, and emotions. Sometimes, I find it helpful to take a step back and simply acknowledge:

Stress and joy are both part of our vast human experience.

Chapter 6

Vulnerability as a Virtue

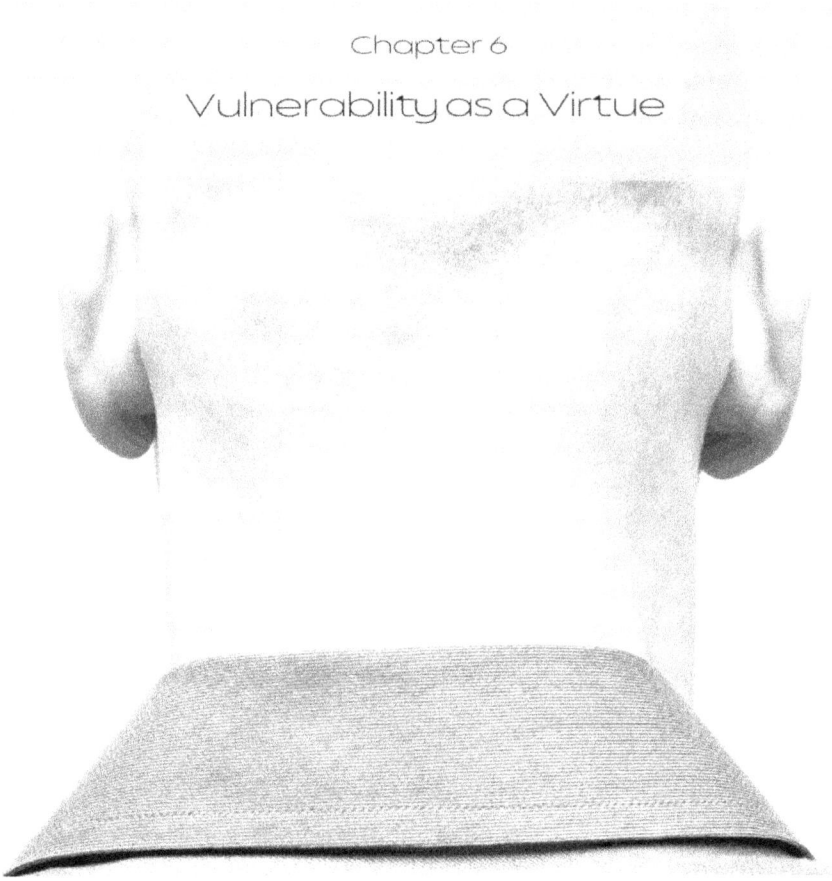

Standing in the softly lit lobby of my yoga studio, I could hear the gentle hum of conversation. The familiar scent of incense wafted around, and the calming palette of the walls provided an ambience that most would find serene.

To many, I am a figure of strength and calm — a seasoned yoga instructor, about to lead a class into an hour of mindfulness and physical discipline. But as I stand there, there's a tremor of nerves, an itch of unease. I do this nearly every day, yet every day I feel that flutter in my stomach, that tightening in my throat.

In an almost ritualistic manner, I walk to the entrance and step outside for a moment. The world seems bigger outside the confines of the studio, and as I draw in a breath, I'm filled with both the vastness of the universe and the acute intensity of my own existence. I remind myself of what my trainer once said, **"Being nervous means that you care."** And I do care. Immensely. Yet, it feels vulnerable, exposed.

Leading a yoga session is more than just teaching postures. It's about being seen, being heard, and allowing oneself to be judged by every eye in the room. Here's my little secret: as much as I love what I do, I often dread that visibility, that scrutiny.

But, in that rawness, in that vulnerability, there's a transformation — a metamorphosis of spirit. When I embrace this vulnerability, I not only empower myself but also uplift everyone around me. This, I've realized, is my truth with alopecia too. Being thrust into the unrelenting limelight, grappling with the loss of something that society often equates with beauty, and fighting the inner demons of self-worth.

But here's the thing: just as with my yoga sessions, if you engage with this vulnerability, if you truly lean into it, there's immense power waiting on the other side. A force that can reshape not just how you see yourself, but how the world sees you.

There was a time, not so long ago, when the very idea of stepping into a yoga studio was a monumental challenge for me. I would sign up for classes, driven by an inner longing, only to find myself paralyzed by an inexplicable fear when the day of the class arrived. I'd stare at my yoga mat, willing myself to go, but my feet felt cemented to the ground. I would make excuses — it's too cold, I'm too tired, maybe next time — but deep down, I knew the truth. It wasn't the cold or fatigue. It was the raw vulnerability of being seen, of being judged, and perhaps, of not measuring up.

I missed several classes, watched numerous opportunities slip by, all because of this invisible wall of resistance. But then, as with all things, the universe conspired. One day, through a combination of sheer will and a sprinkle of serendipity, I walked through the doors of a yoga studio. The air was thick with incense, and the muted sounds of gentle breathing provided a backdrop. There, amidst the calm, I felt the storm of my anxieties subside. The instructor's voice, the harmonious rhythm of synchronized movements, the sense of community — it was as if I'd found a haven, I never knew I needed.

I tried different studios, each with its distinct flavor and aura, until I stumbled upon the one that felt like home. A space where judgment was replaced with understanding, and where every individual, irrespective of their journey, was embraced.

Fast forward a decade, and yoga is no longer just a practice; it's a pillar of my life. The mat has become a reflection of my soul, a space of self-discovery and growth. I often think back to those days of hesitancy and realize that behind that towering wall of resistance was a realm of untapped possibilities. It was my vulnerability, the fear of being seen, that almost robbed me of this transformative journey.

Every wall we encounter, every hurdle that seems insurmountable, is often guarding a treasure of opportunities. The key lies in pushing past that discomfort, embracing the vulnerability, and taking that first step towards what could potentially redefine our lives.

In our journey towards embracing vulnerability, it's essential to recognize its many facets. Vulnerability isn't a singular emotion or state; it's a complex interplay of various fears, hesitations, and insecurities. By identifying and understanding each of these "faces," we are better equipped to confront them head-on. The following list seeks to unravel the diverse aspects of vulnerability we often encounter. By shedding light on them and providing ways to show up for each, we hope to offer you tools to navigate these waters with increased resilience and awareness.

1. Fear of Rejection

How to Show Up: Accept that not everyone will understand or embrace your journey. Seek out supportive communities and remind yourself that your worth isn't determined by external validation.

2. Fear of Being Judged

How to Show Up: Understand that everyone has their own battles and insecurities. Most judgments are reflections of the judger's inner world. Practice self-compassion and embrace self-awareness.

3. Fear of Failure

How to Show Up: Remind yourself that every setback is a set-up for a comeback. Failure is a stepping stone to success and growth. Celebrate the lessons each experience provides.

4. Fear of Being Seen (in your raw, unfiltered state)

How to Show Up: Remember that authenticity resonates. By allowing yourself to be seen in your genuine state, you inspire others to do the same.

5. Overwhelming Shame (from past actions or experiences)

How to Show Up: Understand that everyone has moments they aren't proud of. Embrace forgiveness, both for yourself and others. Seek professional help if the shame feels too heavy.

6. Feeling Inadequate

How to Show Up: Engage in positive self-talk. List out your strengths and achievements. Understand that everyone is at a different point in their journey, and comparison is the thief of joy.

7. Fear of Abandonment

How to Show Up: Nurture strong, deep connections with those who value and understand you. Remember that you are deserving of love and belonging.

8. Fear of the Unknown

How to Show Up: Embrace the present moment. Remember that uncertainty is a part of life, and often, the most beautiful experiences lie beyond the horizon of the unknown.

9. Fear of Being Hurt (emotionally or physically)

How to Show Up: Set boundaries that protect your emotional and physical well-being. Communicate your feelings and needs clearly with those around you.

10. Overexposure (feeling too seen or oversharing)

How to Show Up: It's okay to pull back and take time for yourself. Recognize your boundaries and ensure you're sharing in spaces that feel safe and supportive.

Facing vulnerability requires courage. By acknowledging these faces and understanding how to confront them, we empower ourselves to live more authentically and create deeper connections with others.

Has the sinking feeling of losing your hair felt like the most substantial weight you've ever had to bear? Have those initial moments of realization, coupled with the introspection, placed you at the peak of vulnerability? If they have, then let's pause and reflect for a moment.

Remember the simpler things that used to make you nervous or hesitant? That neighbor you've been meaning to greet, but always found a reason not to? Those casual social interactions that somehow felt like climbing a mountain? When you think about it in perspective, they might now seem like mere molehills compared to the Everest of emotions you're currently scaling.

Hair loss has the potential to redefine your thresholds. What used to be monumental challenges can start to look like easy tasks when placed beside the daunting journey of coming to terms with a changing appearance.

Here's a thought. If facing alopecia has become your biggest vulnerability, then in many ways, it's also your strength. **You're being chiseled and shaped by this experience**. And as the days go by, you'll find that many of the smaller fears, the minor hesitations, begin to fade in its shadow.

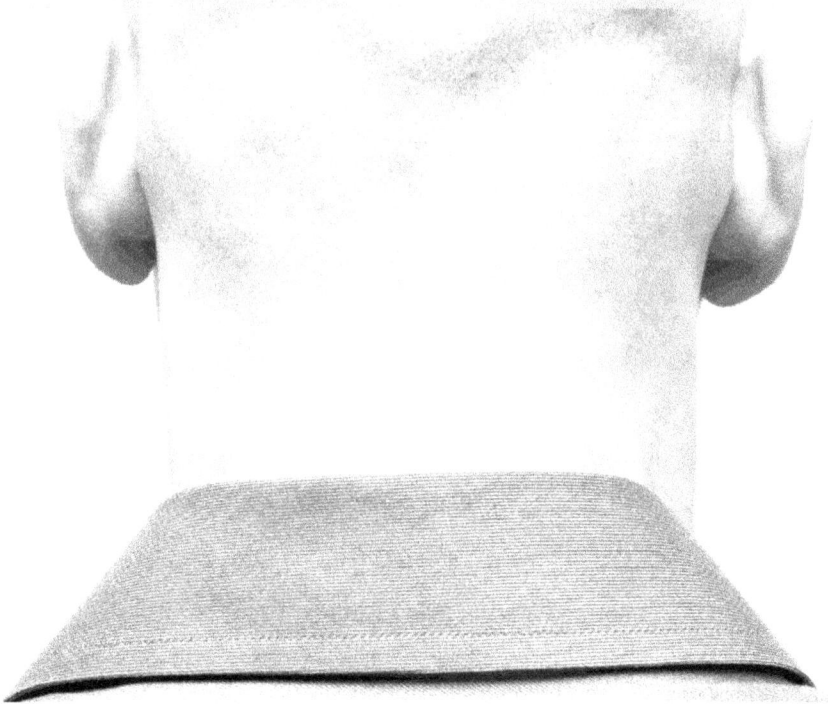

Chapter 7

Pause... Coexist

Breathe. Let's take a moment. Just... pause.

I want to acknowledge that some of you might be reading this with skepticism, with disagreement, perhaps even with a clenched fist. Hey, it's okay. And thanks for sticking around despite the resistance you might be feeling.

You see, I'm not writing this to dictate your emotions or to tell you how you should feel about your journey. It's about sharing, resonating, and understanding. If something doesn't sit right with you, that's valid. Your feelings are valid. If you feel like experiencing alopecia sucks and nothing good can come of it, then that's true for you. No one's denying you that opinion.

What's essential is not whether you agree or disagree with me. It's the journey you're on and the lessons you'll extract from it. There's no magic wand, no one-size-fits-all solution. The experiences, strengths, and growth I share about are true for many, including myself. And I believe they hold true for you too.

Here's a bit of raw truth: **If I could, I'd grow my hair back.** Even after all these years, even though I'm comfortable in my skin, if someone handed me a mystical elixir that would grant me a full head of hair, I'd take a sip without hesitation. Why? Because I still want hair. My answer isn't negating the insights or denying the personal growth that I've encountered on this path. But at the core of it, a part of me still yearns for what once was. And you know what? That's alright.

Every once in a while, it stings. The twinge of longing, the faint whisper of envy, the occasional 'why me?' moments; **they're all real.** They don't detract from the journey, nor do they negate the strengths developed. **They coexist.**

As we continue this journey, it's essential to recognize: life is not about seeking absolute agreement with every perspective or experience. It's about embracing the full spectrum of our emotions and circumstances—the yearning and the acceptance, the **joy** and the **sorrow**. Both paths can and do coexist. By navigating through the highs and the lows, we learn, grow, and emerge stronger.

By fully embracing each experience, we tap into the boundless wellspring of our resilience and savor the multifaceted richness of life.

Chapter 8

The Quest for Regrowth

As we venture on this journey, it's natural to entertain the idea of finding a way back, a path that might restore what once was. The longing for our hair is real, and the quest to regrow it is a path many of us have trodden, including myself.

First and foremost, it's essential to clarify that this book isn't about medical advice. It's not a prescription, nor is it a guide to regrowing your hair. This is a narrative of empathy, understanding, and walking the path together. However, it would be an oversight to not mention the myriad options available to people looking for ways to combat hair loss.

There are countless treatments, regimes, and strategies out there, each promising a solution to the challenges of alopecia and other auto-immune disorders. From dietary changes to curb inflammation to medical treatments, holistic approaches, and even surgical procedures - the landscape is vast and varied.

Why am I telling you this?

Because I want you to know that options exist. I want you to be empowered by knowledge. But here's the crucial point: **I'm not selling hope**. While these treatments might offer potential solutions, it's essential to approach them with a balanced mindset. Every person's journey is unique, and what works for one might not work for another.

During my personal quest to regrow my hair, I explored various avenues. My head is still soft and shiny, but the journey has led me to unexpected rewards. My exploration into anti-inflammatory diets introduced me to healthier eating habits. And although I didn't regain my hair, the path I walked made me a healthier, more aware individual.

The Empowering Side-Effect

In searching for a 'cure' or a solution, there's an unspoken gift - the journey itself. In my quest for hair regrowth, not only did I learn about my body and its reactions, but I also embraced healthier habits, which has left an indelible mark on my overall well-being. You might start a certain diet to curb hair loss, but in the process, find a better version of yourself, physically and mentally.

So, if you're inclined, dive deep, do your research, and explore the avenues available to you. Understand the options, weigh them, and make an informed choice. Regardless of the outcome, remember that every step you take adds to your story, to your growth. And sometimes, the quest itself is more transformative than the destination.

The Many Paths to Explore

While the journey of self-acceptance and empowerment remains at the heart of our narrative, it's equally important to be informed about the various treatments and strategies that many have explored in their bid to tackle hair loss. Let's take a brief look at some popular options:

Autoimmune Protocol Diet (AIP):

This is an elimination and reintroduction diet that aims to reduce inflammation in the body, believed by some to help manage autoimmune conditions, including alopecia.

Steroids:

Injections, creams, and oral steroids can be prescribed to suppress the immune system and prevent it from attacking hair follicles. These treatments might help in certain cases but come with potential side effects.

Ointments and Topical Solutions:

Various over-the-counter and prescription ointments and solutions, such as minoxidil, have been explored by many to promote hair growth.

Acupuncture:

An ancient Chinese practice, acupuncture involves inserting thin needles into specific points on the body. Some believe it can stimulate hair growth by improving blood circulation to the hair follicles.

Meditation:

Chronic stress has been linked to hair loss in some studies. Meditation can be a way to manage stress and promote overall well-being, potentially supporting hair health indirectly.

Yoga:

Like meditation, yoga can be a holistic approach to managing stress and improving circulation. While direct links to hair regrowth are anecdotal, many find solace and strength in the practice.

Hair Transplantation:

This is a surgical procedure where hair follicles from one part of the body are transplanted to areas with no or thinning hair. It's a more permanent solution but requires a thorough evaluation.

Laser Therapy:

Low-level laser therapy is believed to enhance blood flow and stimulate hair follicles. Devices like laser combs and helmets have been designed for this purpose.

Natural Oils and Herbs:

Many swear by the power of natural solutions like rosemary oil, lavender oil, and saw palmetto for promoting hair growth.

PRP (Platelet-Rich Plasma) Treatment:

This involves drawing a person's blood, processing it to isolate the plasma rich in platelets, and injecting it into the scalp. It's believed to foster a healthier environment for hair growth.

It's paramount to note that while numerous paths to treatment and understanding alopecia exist, their efficacy can differ from one individual to the next. The exploration of these paths can often lead to broader discoveries about oneself and one's health. Whether you find success in regrowth or discover new aspects of your well-being, remember that every journey is valuable.

However, in a world where information is abundant, it's also a haven for misinformation. Books, websites, and influencers might guarantee miraculous results, often with a hidden agenda or product to sell. While the promise of a quick fix is tempting, it's crucial to remember that real solutions are typically backed by science and medical expertise. Always consult with a healthcare professional before diving into a new treatment or remedy.

Currently, certain drugs have shown promise in clinical trials, but a one-size-fits-all cure remains beyond our grasp. Our hope is that one day such a cure will be within reach. Until that day, let's cherish our journey, embrace our truths, and always **prioritize our well-being.**

Chapter 9

The Abyss and the Beacon

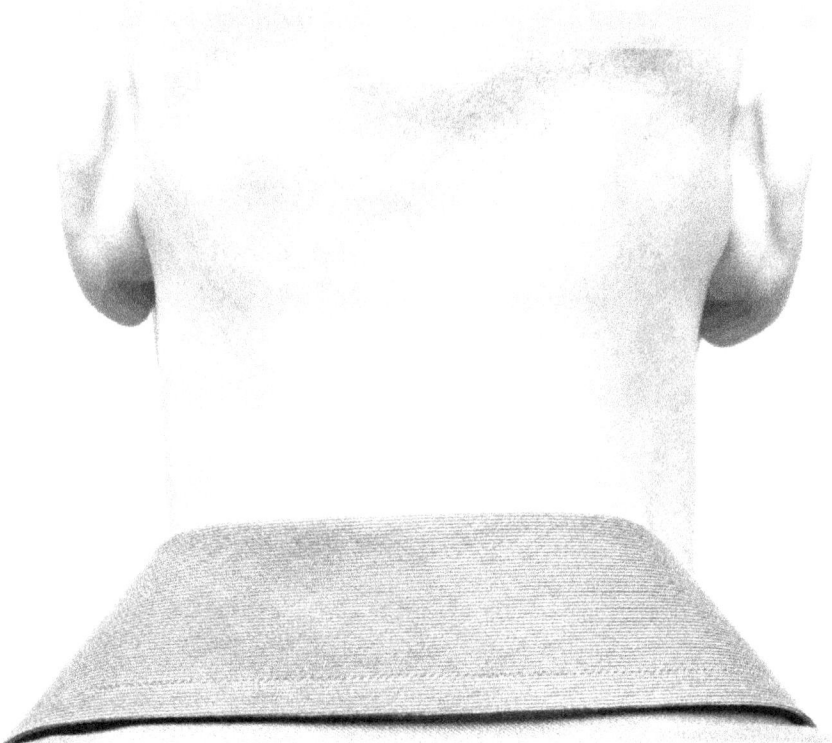

Important note Before You Continue: This chapter contains references to personal despair and an attempt at self-harm. Please proceed with caution if these topics might be triggering for you. Your well-being is important. If you or someone you know is struggling, please consider seeking professional help or reaching out to a trusted individual in your life.

It's easy to gloss over the brighter sides of a journey, to share uplifting anecdotes and offer a silver lining. But sometimes, the journey to self-acceptance takes us to dark, haunting places where despair feels unending. It's essential to shed light on these moments, to ensure that anyone navigating such despair knows they're not alone.

There I was, fourteen years old, lying in the cold embrace of a bathtub, water faded from comforting warmth to chilling indifference. With a bald head, fresh from the razor, every ounce of my being felt trapped, suffocated, as if a thousand-pound weight pressed on my chest.

What does one think in those moments? Of life's cruelty, the unfairness of it all, or simply a desperate wish to escape the inescapable. My train of thought was interrupted when I tried, in a fleeting act of despair, to inhale water instead of air. Pain, coughing, the sharp reality of survival instincts kicked in, and there I was, sprawled on cold tiles, clutching a towel around me, gasping for breath.

The door burst open, and my mom rushed in. Her face, a mixture of concern, love, and fear, mirrored my own feelings. What transpired in those moments, the words shared, the pain acknowledged, has since become a guiding light in my life.

"Everyone has their thing," she began, her voice soft yet firm. "Yours might be baldness, but everyone carries something. A burden, a regret, a shadow. It could be their weight, appearance, an injury, a failed relationship, an addiction... something."

What she said next that truly pierced through my anguish, **"When you hurt, I hurt."** Simple words, yet they echoed with profound truth. In those words, I felt the world's weight lift slightly. There was no judgment, no attempt to diminish my pain. Just pure, unfiltered empathy.

Empathy is a powerful tool. It's not just about understanding someone else's pain, but truly feeling it. Even now, writing these words, I'm echoing that sentiment to you, whoever you may be, wherever you're reading this. If you're in pain, know that you're not alone. Every word on this page, every anecdote and piece of advice, is rooted in empathy. This book's existence has been forged years ago amid deep pain. We may be in different places, on different timelines, but **we are in this together.**

It's challenging to find purpose or even a sliver of hope in such darkness, but if this chapter achieves one thing, I hope it's this: to anyone teetering on the edge, take a deep breath, not of water, but of air. There's a world of understanding, support, and genuine empathy waiting for you.

My mother's wisdom, shared with me during one of the most pivotal moments in my life, didn't just offer solace in that fleeting instance. It planted a seed. A seed that, over time, blossomed into a profound understanding of empathy, compassion, and the interconnectedness of our human experience.

As I move forward in my journey and imagine the potential of bringing a new life into this world, the significance of passing on these invaluable lessons to future generations becomes abundantly clear. If I ever have children, they will undoubtedly face their own unique challenges, as we all do. But one thing I am determined to instill in them is the power of empathy, the strength in understanding and truly feeling another person's pain.

By doing so, they won't just navigate their struggles with more resilience and grace; they'll become beacons of hope for others. They'll be equipped with the tools to not just soothe their own wounds but also to comfort and uplift those around them.

It's not just about the words we say or the advice we give. Empathy is a language of the heart. It's in the silent moments when we sit beside someone, sharing in their sorrow, without trying to change or fix anything. It's in the act of listening, deeply and intently, validating another's feelings without judgment.

To you, dear reader, I want to extend an invitation…

When someone shares empathy with you, don't just let it wash over you. Absorb it. Internalize it. Let it resonate in your being. And then, when the time is right, pay it forward. Take those feelings, those words of solace and understanding, and echo them to someone else in need. **Become a conduit of compassion, a bridge between pain and solace.**

Through this, we create a beautiful cycle. The lessons we learn will not just remain with us. They will reverberate through time, touching lives and mending hearts for generations to come.

In embracing empathy, we not only heal ourselves, but we also ensure that the world around us becomes a kinder, more compassionate place. Let us all strive to be links in this chain of understanding, binding us all in the shared experience of our humanity.

In our journey through life, challenges like bullying, personal despair, or feelings of isolation can sometimes become overwhelming. Your mental and emotional health is paramount. There's strength in seeking support and understanding. If you, or someone you know, are facing challenges, please remember:

You're not alone: Many before you have walked similar paths, faced similar struggles, and have found ways to cope, heal, and thrive.

Seeking help is a sign of strength: It's not an admission of defeat but a recognition of the courage it takes to share your feelings and vulnerabilities.

Resources are available: From helplines and counseling services to support groups, there's a world of understanding and assistance waiting for you. Always remember that there's strength in unity and healing in understanding.

Chapter 10

The Invisible Threads of Empathy

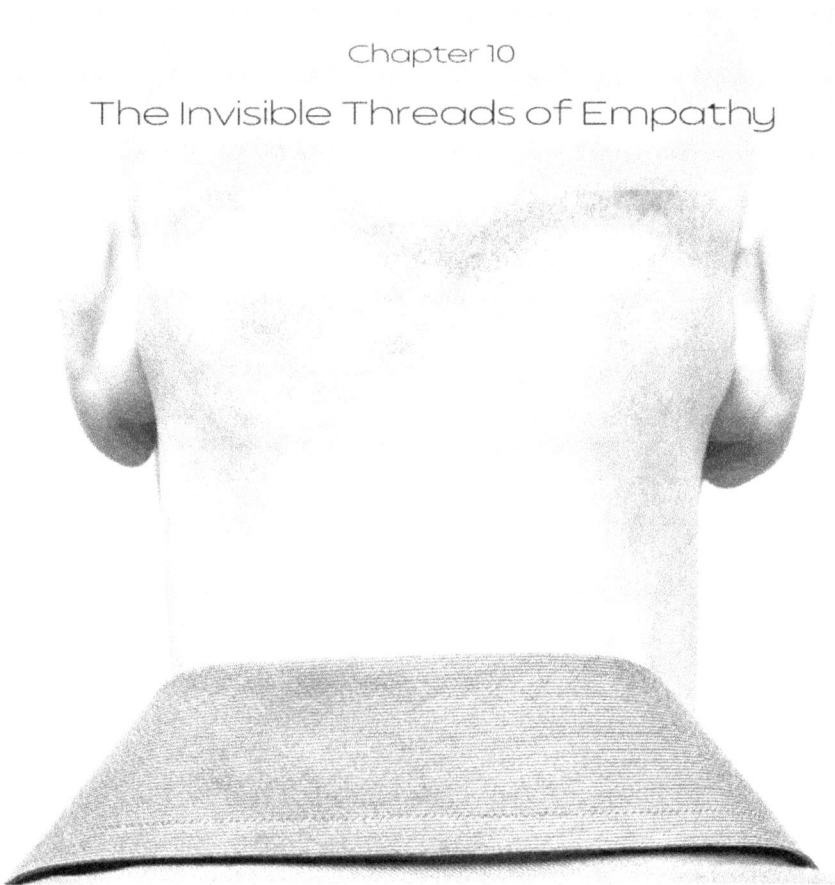

Every journey has its unexpected treasures—moments that stand out, teaching us things we hadn't planned to learn but which end up being profoundly meaningful. When I began my journey into vulnerability, stemming from my own struggle with hair loss, I never expected it to lead me to become someone to whom people easily opened up. But it did, in ways that continue to astonish me.

There I was, standing outside my college classroom, cigarette in hand—a habit I've since quit and strongly advise against. I was minding my own business in the designated smoking area when a young woman, about my age, approached me and timidly said hello. Within moments, tears were streaming down her face.

We sat down, and she began pouring out her soul, sharing the abusive relationship she was in. I listened. I didn't judge. I checked in to ensure she was safe, convinced that she was or would seek the help she needed if she wasn't. She wasn't looking for a savior; she was seeking a listener. We finished our cigarettes, shared a moment of silence, and went our separate ways. We'd see each other around campus, exchange nods, but never more. Nothing else was required.

The Gift of Listening

I can't say for certain why she chose to share with me, a stranger. But I suspect it has something to do with the invisible threads of empathy that connect us. I wasn't there to fix her, to give advice, or to judge. I was just there, being openly human in my own vulnerability, and that made a difference. I had become a person who people felt comfortable opening up to, and that power, my friends, is enormous.

The Ripple Effect

This wasn't an isolated experience; it's happened many times, in various settings, some more unexpected than others. Whether at a rowdy party where someone leans in and admits, "I was depressed for years," or other scenarios where people open up to share their 'thing,' the theme remains consistent. My baldness, lack of eyebrows, and eyelashes might serve as subtle signals that say, "This soul knows pain too," or it might just be the general aura of empathy. Regardless, people seem to feel safe sharing with me, and I consider that a reward and a responsibility.

Embrace and Ponder

I have no empirical data to suggest that this experience is unique to me or those who have faced similar challenges. But the frequency with which it occurs makes me stop and think. Is it that others sense an unspoken understanding? That they intuitively recognize the mask and vulnerability I wear not as a disguise, but as an invitation to mutual humanity?

Whatever it is, one thing is certain: there's incredible power in being someone to whom others can bare their souls. This power is neither a gift nor a curse; it's a responsibility—one that has made my journey into vulnerability all the more worthwhile.

As we continue to navigate the path of empathy, let us be aware of our own vulnerabilities and how they can forge unexpected connections. It's in these connections that we find the extraordinary potential to not just heal ourselves but to offer the priceless gift of a listening ear to others.

Note to the Reader:

As we travel through life, we pick up habits—some beneficial, others detrimental. Smoking was one of those habits for me. I won't romanticize it, but I won't shy away from it either. It was a part of my journey, as were the lessons learned from it.

Research indicates that smoking can exacerbate conditions like alopecia and certainly does no favors for overall well-being. It's a path I've since departed from, for both health and personal reasons. **The key is awareness and making choices that align with our better selves.** If you're grappling with habits or situations that aren't serving your best interests, remember that **seeking help**, whether for wellness or mental peace, **is both brave and essential**.

In this book, as in life, I aim to share the real, the raw, and the authentic—not as endorsements, but as touchpoints of a journey that, like all journeys, has its share of mistakes, learnings, and growth.

Chapter 11

Moving Forward - A Journey of Purpose

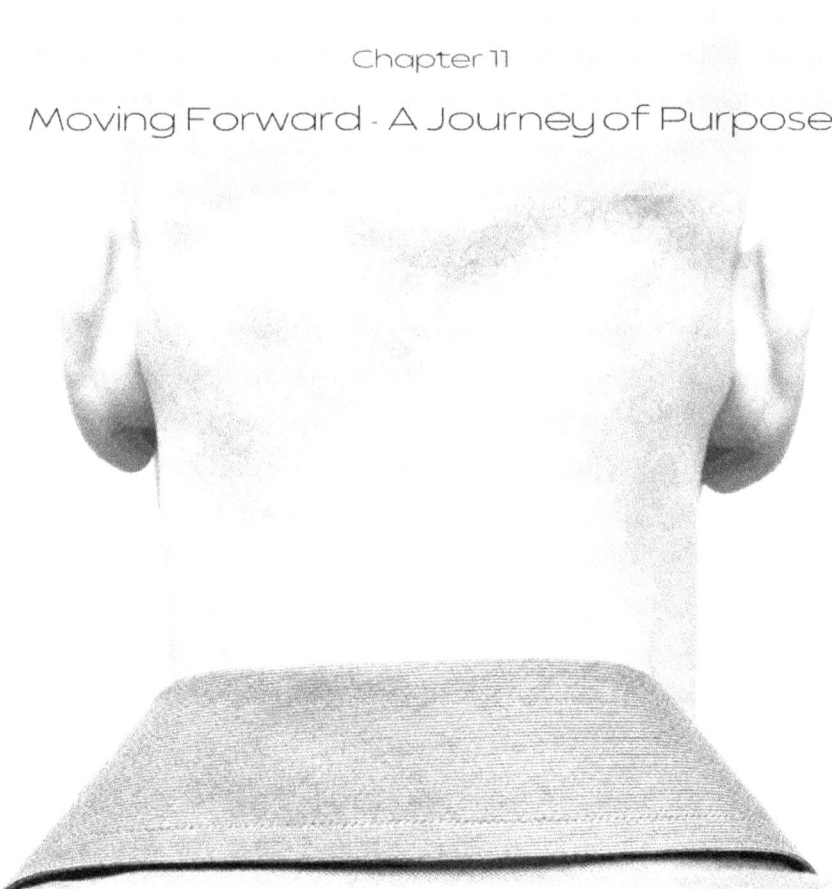

Facing challenges, like hair loss, can knock us down in ways we never anticipated. However, it's the journey through the storm that helps us build resilience, find empathy, and shape our characters. But how do we keep this momentum? What can we do to channel these experiences and insights into positive actions?

Today: Self-awareness and Acceptance

Self-reflection: Spend some time contemplating your experiences, feelings, and learnings. Write them down in a journal, talk to someone about them, or simply ponder while taking a walk.

Acknowledge your feelings: Allow yourself to feel—whether it's anger, sadness, or acceptance. Recognize these emotions without judgment. This is your journey, and every emotion is valid.

Tomorrow: Reach Out and Connect

Share your story: Whether it's with friends, family, or on a platform, let others in. Your story might resonate with someone going through a similar experience.

Connect with others: Join support groups, online forums, or local community events. These platforms can provide not only support but also give you a chance to support others.

Moving Forward: Turning Insights into Actions

Cultivate gratitude: Everyday, find something to be thankful for. This practice helps shift the focus from what we lack to what we have.

Keep learning:

Dive deeper into understanding the science, psychology, or stories related to your experiences. Equip yourself with knowledge.

Advocate:

Use your experiences to make a difference. It could be by raising awareness, supporting research, or just being there for someone else going through a tough time.

The Bigger Picture: Why Does This Matter?

Moving forward with purpose isn't just about personal growth. It's about harnessing the collective power of shared experiences to make a tangible difference in the world. Every step you take, no matter how small, adds up to create a ripple effect that can touch countless lives. By embracing your journey and using it as a catalyst for positive change, you contribute to a world where vulnerability becomes strength, where challenges morph into opportunities, and where every individual, regardless of their 'thing', feels seen, heard, and valued.

In my journey, both through the teachings I've absorbed and the life I've lived, I've come to perceive a universal truth: **we, as humans, are often oscillating between the pursuit of pleasure and the quest for purpose.** I've tasted the joys of pleasures, and I've immersed myself in fulfillment derived from purpose. It's become evident to me that while pleasures are transient, flickering momentarily, purpose has the capacity to transcend, to grow, to become something far bigger than ourselves. **It's the pursuit of purpose that carves out a life of significance, shaping not only our existence but also the world around us.**

Choosing purpose is an act of strength and transformation. It's the courageous decision to see beyond fleeting desires and to find meaning in the mundane, the painful, and the unexpected. You have the power to choose purpose out of your experiences, to see your journey as a vessel for deeper understanding and larger truths.

And choosing purpose is not a one-time act; it's a series of deliberate, mindful decisions made every day, every moment. It's in the quiet resilience after every fall, the silent commitment to growth amidst despair. And as you traverse this journey, remember, every challenge overcome is not just a victory but a beacon of hope, a testament to human spirit and its boundless capacity to evolve and inspire.

Once you've conquered the mountain before you—and conquer it, you will—the wisdom and strength you've amassed will illuminate every challenge that follows. Every hurdle, every obstacle will then become an opportunity, a path to seek and serve a bigger, more profound purpose.

Facing challenges isn't about navigating through pain to reach pleasure; it's about transforming pain into purpose, about realizing that the depth of our struggles can be the wellspring of our greatest contributions to the world. It's about recognizing that in the pursuit of purpose, we find the most enduring, the most enriching form of pleasure—the pleasure derived from growth, contribution, and connection.

As you move forward, let the choices you make be imbued with purpose, let your actions echo with the wisdom of your journey, and let every step you take be a catalyst for change, compassion, and collective awakening. By choosing purpose, by transforming our vulnerabilities into virtues, we don't just enrich our lives; we become architects of a world where every heart knows its worth, every soul recognizes its potential, and every being can choose a life of purpose over fleeting pleasures.

Gandhi once proclaimed,

"Be the change that you wish to see in the world."

He never implied it would be a simple task.

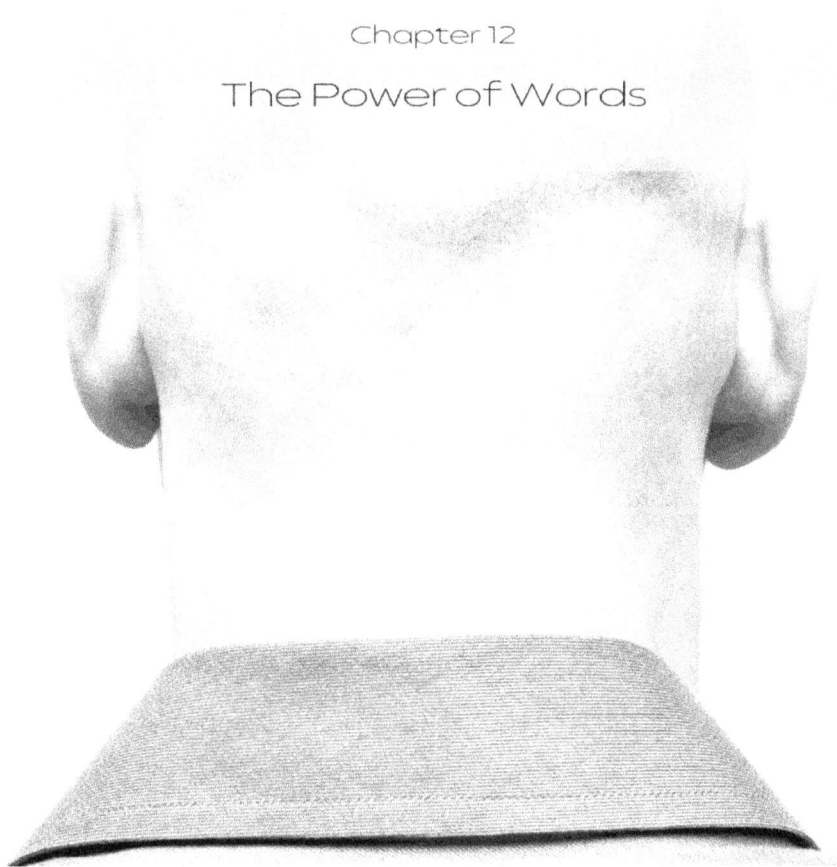

Chapter 12

The Power of Words

Our lives are composed of moments, both dark and bright. There are days when even the strongest among us need a beacon to guide us through the storm. For me, that beacon often took the form of words – simple, profound quotes that resonated deeply with my experiences.

During one of the most challenging phases of my life, I chanced upon a quote that sat on my desk, a leftover from my predecessor at the ski shop. It read, **"Our greatest glory is not in never falling, but in rising every time we fall."** – Confucius. The mountain shaped sticker that housed the quote seemed intended to inspire resilience in skiing. I found solace in these words during the turbulent times at my job and in my personal life.

Despite the quote's seemingly simplistic nature, its profound meaning transformed my perspective. Every time I felt defeated, every time I felt like I had lost my way, I'd look at these words, and they'd remind me of my strength, my capacity to bounce back. This powerful experience led me on a journey to discover more such words that inspire and uplift.

Over the years, I've accumulated a treasure trove of quotes that have held my hand during tough times and cheered me on during my best. Here's a list of a few that I've found incredibly empowering:

"To **be yourself** in a world that is constantly trying to make you something else is the **greatest accomplishment**."
 - Ralph Waldo Emerson

"Our life is what our thoughts make it." - Marcus Aurelius

"In the middle of every difficulty lies opportunity."
- Albert Einstein

"I am not afraid of storms, for I am learning how to sail my ship."
 - Louisa May Alcott

"He who has a *why* to live can bear almost any *how*."
  - Friedrich Nietzsche

"Life isn't about finding yourself. Life is about **creating yourself**."
 - George Bernard Shaw

"Act as if what you do makes a difference. **It does**."
 - William James

Each of these quotes holds a story, an essence, and a promise. They remind us that life's challenges, though overwhelming at times, also bring growth, wisdom, and a renewed spirit. And there are so many more incredible quotes out there! Every day, I try to find a new quote that uplifts me, and I encourage us all to do the same. Let's surround with these beacons of hope and let them light our path.

Before I share this next quote, I'd like to offer some context. It's my favorite quote, the one I'd like to leave you with. This passage comes from Theodore Roosevelt's speech, "Citizenship in a Republic," which he delivered at the Sorbonne in Paris in 1910. I've taken the liberty of adapting it to be non-binary, with the intent of ensuring it speaks to everyone. By making these alterations, I mean absolutely no disrespect to Teddy. In fact, Theodore Roosevelt is one of my personal role models. His impact on the world, as I've come to understand it, inspires me to keep striving to reach my fullest potential.

"It is not the critic who counts; not the person who points out how the strong one stumbles, or where the doer of deeds could have done them better. The credit belongs to the person who is actually in the arena, whose face is marred by dust and sweat and blood; who strives valiantly; who errs, who comes short again and again, because there is no effort without error and shortcoming; but who does actually strive to do the deeds; who knows great enthusiasms, the great devotions; who spends oneself in a worthy cause; who at the best knows in the end the triumph of high achievement, and who at the worst, if they fail, at least fails while daring greatly, so that their place shall never be with those cold and timid souls who neither know victory nor defeat."

- Theodore Roosevelt

After soaking in the wisdom of others through their quotes, I began to contemplate the power of our own words, especially the ones we silently utter to ourselves. The dialogue we maintain with our inner selves is perhaps the most influential and potent conversation we engage in daily.

You see, the words we choose in our thoughts shape our realities. It is through this internal discourse that we either empower or disempower ourselves. Each thought acts as a brushstroke, painting the canvas of our lives. And like any artist, the colors we choose – be they dark or bright – define our masterpiece.

How often have you caught yourself in a loop of negative self-talk? Reprimanding yourself for past mistakes, doubting your capabilities, or chastising yourself for perceived imperfections. But here's the catch: when you're the bully in your own mind, you're both the perpetrator and the victim. The harm is twofold.

It's oddly tempting to fall into this pattern, isn't it? There's an almost addictive quality to self-deprecation. It feels good to play the disciplinarian, to set high standards, to be the critic. But this fleeting satisfaction comes at a hefty price. When we constantly belittle ourselves, we diminish our self-worth, stunt our growth, and undermine our potential.

It's essential to remember that every word, every thought, carries weight. **If we wouldn't say it to someone we love, why would we say it to ourselves?** Kindness, patience, and compassion should not only be reserved for others but also extended generously to ourselves. Switching from negative to positive self-talk doesn't happen overnight. It requires a conscious effort, a deliberate reprogramming of the mind. Start by challenging those self-deprecating thoughts. Question their validity. Counter them with positive affirmations.

For those navigating the emotional landscape of alopecia, the journey is complex and at times, overwhelmingly challenging. It's all too easy for us to spiral into self-criticism. Thoughts like, "I'm not attractive anymore," or "People are judging me," might cloud our minds. Even when armed with knowledge and insight, resistance can still rear its head. It's natural to have moments of doubt, pain, and longing for what once was.

Amidst this tumultuous journey, there's room for reframing. Instead of lamenting, "Why is this happening to me?" we might ponder, **"How can we use this experience to grow stronger?"** Rather than resigning with, "I miss the old me," empower ourselves with, **"I am evolving, and every version of me has its own beauty."**

Our mind is like fertile soil. And especially when dealing with alopecia, it's vital to sow seeds of self-compassion and resilience. While it's okay to grieve and feel the weight of your situation, it's equally crucial to nurture positive affirmations. The thoughts you care for today will shape your perceptions, attitudes, and actions tomorrow. Yes, the road might be tough, but why not cultivate a mindset where you're your own most significant source of encouragement and hope?

Buddha once said, **"What we think, we become."** Think with kindness, embrace every phase of your journey with positivity, and be patient with yourself when times are tough. The journey, with all its twists and turns, holds lessons and transformations that only you can uniquely experience and share.

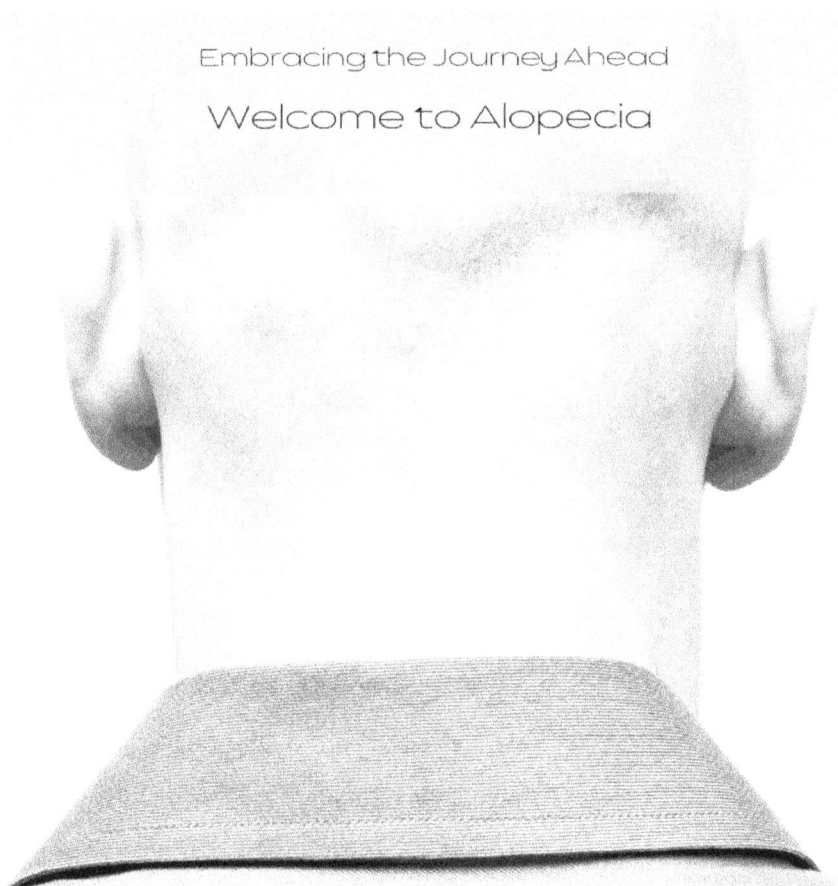

Embracing the Journey Ahead

Welcome to Alopecia

In the journey of life, sometimes the path isn't what we expect it to be. It's filled with twists, turns, valleys, and peaks. It's a tapestry of emotions, experiences, and revelations. This journey of alopecia is no different. So, as we reach the close of this book, I wish to truly welcome you to alopecia…

Welcome to the strength you never knew you had. The strength to face the world with a balding head, patchy beard, no eyebrows, or no eyelashes, and to still stand tall. The strength to embrace your true self, to accept, and to love unconditionally.

Welcome to the empathy that will become a part of your core. As you've learned through my experiences and perhaps your own, people will open up to you, sharing their vulnerabilities. Because, like you, they too have their 'thing'. In this shared understanding, we find a collective strength.

Welcome to the journey of self-discovery. From the depths of despair in a cold bathtub to the heights of self-realization in a yoga studio, the journey is filled with moments of darkness and light. It's about understanding that while our physical appearance might change, our essence undergoes an evolution. With each experience, it molds and shifts, and in this self-discovery and acknowledgment lies the power to guide and embrace that transformation.

Welcome to a community. Yes, Alopecia isn't just a condition; it's a community. A community of brave souls, facing similar challenges, supporting each other, and reminding one another that they aren't alone in this journey.

Welcome to the wisdom of ages. Through quotes, through stories, through shared experiences, we gain insights from thinkers of the past and the present. Let them be your guiding star as you navigate through the challenges ahead.

Lastly, **welcome to a life filled with potential and purpose.**

Your alopecia isn't a flaw; it's a feature. It's a part of the story, a chapter in the book of life, but it's not the entirety. As Theodore Roosevelt said, "It's not the critic who counts..." Remember, it's about daring greatly, even when faced with adversity.

In this book, we've traveled together through the landscapes of emotions, challenges, and revelations. As you move forward, remember that Alopecia isn't just a condition; it's an invitation—

An invitation to discover your inner strength, to connect deeply with others, to live authentically, and to inspire those around you.

So, with arms wide open, heart full of empathy, and spirit soaring high, I say to you once more - **Welcome to Alopecia**. Embrace your journey, for it promises growth, wisdom, and a renewed spirit. Embrace every part of yourself and, in doing so, illuminate the world around you.

Own your story and be the radiant badass the world needs.

Dear Reader,

From the depth of my heart, I thank you for joining me on this journey. This book, while rooted in my own experiences with alopecia, is as much yours as it is mine. It's about our shared struggles, our battles with acceptance, and our steps towards self-love.

Your choice to pick up "Welcome to Alopecia." and immerse yourself in its pages is a testament to your strength and the beginning of a beautiful dialogue we now share. Every story is powerful, and I am deeply honored that you allowed mine to intertwine with yours, even if just for a little while.

I hope these words offer comfort, inspiration, and a sense of camaraderie. Remember, you're never alone in your journey.

Lastly, a heartfelt thank you to everyone who's supported, encouraged, and walked beside me throughout this endeavor. This book wouldn't have been possible without the love and support of so many.

Warmly,
Nitka Marga

About
NITKA MARGA

About Nitka Marga

Nitka Marga's writings artfully blend introspection with rich narratives. While he skillfully navigates between light-hearted humor and profound reflections, a consistent thread of positive teachings and personal growth shines through each piece.

Personal Journey

Nitka's resilience and unique perspective on life have been shaped by his personal journey with alopecia. This experience, combined with his roles as a dedicated yoga teacher and entrepreneur, has deeply enriched his path of empowerment and self-discovery. His writing, infused with these personal insights, resonates with themes of self-growth, transformation, and empathy. "Welcome to Alopecia" stands as a testament to this journey, offering a heartfelt guide to those facing the challenges of alopecia and providing understanding for readers looking to deepen their empathy.

About

NITKA MARGA

Diverse Interests

A passionate yogi and advocate for wellness, Nitka masterfully blends ancient philosophies and modern insights into his work. His narratives not only captivate with wisdom and practical insights but also invite readers to embark on their own journey of self-discovery and reflection.

Writing Style

Nitka's stories traverse beyond mere words. They serve as gateways to self-reflection, offering fresh perspectives and timeless truths. Dive into Nitka Marga's world, where humor, wisdom, and introspection come together, shining a light for those navigating the intricacies of human experience.

.

www.ingramcontent.com/pod-product-compliance
Lightning Source LLC
Chambersburg PA
CBHW032049040426

42449CB00007B/1043